How to Excel at Weight Loss and Become More Fit and Healthy

Carol Langkamp

Disclaimer

This book is an authentic story and continuation of the author's weight loss journey. Mention of specific companies, organizations or authorities in this book does not imply endorsement by the author or publisher, not does mention of specific companies, organizations or authorities imply that they endorse this book, its author or the publisher.

Internet addresses given in this book were accurate at the time it went to press.

The author and publisher do not assume and hereby disclaim any liability to any party for any loss, damage, or disruption caused by errors or omissions, whether such errors or omissions result from negligence, accident, or any other cause.

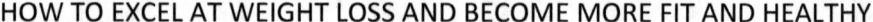

The Clean Plate Club

Are you a member of the clean plate club? Were you told you could not leave the dinner table until your plate was totally clean (empty)? Or were you told your asparagus would be there waiting for you at breakfast?

How many of us were told, "There are starving children in Africa who would die for this meal?"

Then there's also television commercials stating, "It's good to the last drop!" Who says?

Now, don't get me wrong. I believe in conserving our resources and I do recycle. However, I am a product of the "clean plate" mindset. I would never send my food scraps to starving children anywhere in the world. For one thing, the food would not be good or fresh by the time it got there so they would probably die of food poisoning. If you are really worried about starving children in parts of the world, send money or get involved in a local mission or food pantry.

I realize today how much this "clean plate mentality" has influenced me.

As I was fixing my breakfast it occurred to me that I was extremely thirsty. I always keep a variety of water containers in my refrigerator as I love cold water. (Yes, I know bottled spring water is better for you but I still drink from the tap as I can't afford the other.) Anyhow, I grabbed my glass container of water only to realize that it was almost all gone. As I am filling my cup, I find myself thinking, "I can gulp this down and refill it again so the container is empty."

STOP! HOLD UP! Why should I gulp this down and not enjoy it? I am not in any rush or any race. I sat down with my breakfast and water and put the container back in the fridge.

Here is another example.

I am at home with my Mom making muffins. Normally I scrape the bowl with a rubber scraper and get every last little morsel out of the bowl and into the muffin tins. However, it was Mom who was baking, not me. She had scraped the bowl and left some in it. This really bothered me and I thought about pointing it out, but she had already put the bowl in the sink with warm soapy water.

This was not the first time this had happened to me. I've gone through the same exact scenario with my friends when I cook with them. It's as if life depends on getting that last little morsel out of the bowl.

I learned early in life that you need to eat all your food and save everything to reuse and recycle it so that you are not wasting anything. Yet as far as the food goes, you are wasting it because your own waistline is getting bigger and bigger and bigger.

You get my drift? Now, don't get me wrong. I am not blaming my parents; as I love them dearly and know they did the very best they could. I am just pointing out things that I have learned about my food addiction and what helped it prosper and flourish.

I mentioned saving things to recycle them... If you have ever been to my place, you know I have lots of stuff – whether it be books, crafts, toys, games, candles, clothes, notebooks, greeting cards or what else, have you, I definitely have it. I am not a hoarder like the ones you see on television but I definitely need to get rid of some things.

When I was growing up, I remember saving birthday cards, Christmas cards and papers from school. It was atrocious, the stacks of cards, invites, postcards I had when I first moved out on my own. Now, granted, I really appreciate the messages and I enjoy receiving cards but I can't afford to keep them all. Besides, isn't life about interacting with others and enjoying their company? If you constantly have the battle of cleaning out clutter, you are losing valuable time in your life that could be spent enjoying nature or the company of others. Life is short even on the days that drag on and on. It goes faster every day or so it seems.

The older I get, the more important it is to me that I get rid of this clutter. As stated before I waste quality time cleaning and organizing, trying to find a place for all these things. I find myself thinking that people who are minimalists probably enjoy their life more as they have more time to enjoy it! There is more time to travel and socialize when you do not have things all over the place. Plus another thing I realize is that with all this mess I have so much to distract me from focusing on one task and am often off on 5 different tangents without finishing any of the activities I started!

For those of you that may be confused on the relationship between my eating disorder and this issue of too much clutter and stuff, think about it this way. The happier you are, the better you feel. The less happy you are, the more you feel the need to "stuff" yourself to fill the void and fill the emptiness. I believe spending money on material possessions is one of the ways to fill this black hole. No matter how hard you try to fill this emptiness, you get further and further from feeling really happy and satisfied.

Breaking Point and Breaking Free

Confession time... Yes, I have slipped once again. You see, my mindset is when you want to celebrate, you eat. Not just any kind of food but sugar and fat filled junk. That is what celebration means, doesn't it? Or so it seems.

Time to eat...

I reach for food when...

I am overjoyed,

I am mad,

I am sad,

I am lonely,

I am celebrating,

I want something,

I feel empty.

"Life is truly more than becoming rich, finding the love of your life, getting the right job, waking up every morning or even reading a good book. You find when you pursue a life of greater health and happiness; you then **treat the body you have with dignity, respect, and absolute care**."

Dale L. Roberts, page 1 in <u>The 3 Keys to Greater Health & Happiness</u>

So, Now Where Do I Start?

I am feeling empty, hopeless, and heartless. Death may be knocking at my door and in this state I may even welcome it. Is my life worth it? What is love? What is the meaning of my life? I am fat, overweight, obese, addicted to food. I feel as if I have no friends. I am worthless and have no value. I am miserable.

Jobs come and go but nothing appeals to me. I am an average worker and not very successful in finding the right job, whatever it may be. Who am I? Why do I exist? What is my purpose in life? This is the question I really need to answer. Why was I put on this Earth? What should I do with this existence? Why was I placed in this family? Who are they and what role do I play? Do I really have friends? Am I just a failure at everything? In other words, I am just a blob. A sack of sugar... actually several pounds of it.

Whew! Thank God those days are over for me. *****Or are they?**** I no longer wake up and feel like staying in bed all day long. I get up and am grateful for what I do have: a roof over my head, a place to live, a whole body that functions and moves for me, food to eat, clothes to wear, friends that care, family to share.

At this point in my life, I am not sure what tomorrow will bring or

what job I will have but I know that I am in control of my life and

happiness. I have made the choice. I can choose to worry about the

future, I mean, where am I going? How am I getting there and all

the "what ifs" I can imagine. But, thankfully, I have decided I am

living in the moment, the present time is all I have and all I am. The

past has come and gone and I cannot change it, the future is coming

and I am not in control of it other than my present actions that may

or may not affect it. I live everyday thankfully, gratefully to be alive

and to live my life to the best of my abilities. I may not always feel

like eating right and exercising but I know what the consequences

are for those actions. I have lived that life for most of my existence

and it ain't pretty. I want something more. I deserve it. I am worth

it!

Now, I am not saying to give up what you have but I am saying to

take inventory of your life. Are you doing what you want to do? Do

you have dreams or do you have regrets? Do you enjoy what you do for work? Are you just working to please others or are you happy with what you are doing? Yes, I know, not everybody can choose to survive the way I am suggesting but I can tell you this. Somehow, some way, I am surviving. My main focus and the most important goal for me in my life is health driven. My workouts with my trainer are the most important asset in my life and that is what has helped me lose as much weight as I have. Yes, I admit this is not the only thing that has made me successful in losing weight but once I decided this was the most important goal for my life; that is when change started to occur. In the past, I worked out sporadically and tried for years to lose weight, but I was not as committed and driven as I am now. My outlook about life has changed. I used to think, I am such a failure. I mean I thought by the time I was 30, I would be happily married, own a house, have kids, a dog or two, a beautiful yard, a great job or career, travel several times a year. However, most of these things have not happened for me. I have had a dog and have traveled a few times but not as much as I had planned. Also, I love my current employment as a tutor. There have been some other jobs that I have enjoyed but this one takes the cake... sorry for the food reference! Also, I have found I love writing too! You may say, yes, but do I know how my bills are going to get paid and where the money is coming from? The answer is no, I do not but somehow, some way I have found a way to pay for training sessions, gym membership and I am still living in an apartment that I have to pay rent for monthly. I survive. There are ways to make do and there are times that I may not do everything I want but I find I can be happy now, much more so than ever before. I believe in my heart the reason is because I am taking care of my health and making changes for the better, which helps strengthen my self-esteem and wellbeing! It may have taken me half my life to get here, but it is a much better place to live than where I have been in the past.

I would like to share a few words from my mentor and good friend, Dale L.Roberts.

"The three keys of staying active, eating healthfully and building a strong mindset can bring you the much needed success that you may have

always wanted, but never knew where to start. When you implement

these three keys, you discover true happiness."

Excerpt from <u>The 3 Keys to Greater Health & Happiness</u>, page 2.

Food Plan

I need to discuss my food plan or at least what I have learned from working with a variety of trainers over the years. One thing is for sure, you will not lose weight if you keep eating all kinds of crap. It is like the saying, "Garbage in, garbage out." And believe me, this saying tells you how you feel if you survive on junk. I have been there done that and those are my worst days. I feel headachy, sick to my stomach, lethargic and little to no energy to be found. I consider those my "slug days". Slug, because that is about all I accomplish on those days. You may think I have broken the mold for this but it still happens on occasion. Luckily I have learned ways of coping when I feel them coming on and can usually find some way to survive without overindulging. Besides, do you really want those extra chemicals that wreak havoc on your body? I mean think about how prevalent cancer is in our society. It just keeps killing off people and I believe part of the reason for this is the fact that most of our food is processed and filled with chemical preservatives and things to make it taste good, even though they are artificial ingredients.

Needless to say I have been on many different weight loss plans. If you want a recommendation, I can tell you that Dr. Phil McGraw's Ultimate Weight Solution is the one commercialized plan that worked the best for me and that was without any regular exercise too. (I started on this plan the year my Dad died and I lost a total of 50 pounds on his plan within 2 ½ months!) I know he has a new plan but I have not tried it out.

The most recent plan I have been on is one my trainer gave me and I cannot share that with you. However, there are some concepts and facts that I can tell you about right now.

First off, if you are serious and truly want to lose weight, you need to start by cleaning out your kitchen. Get rid of **all** the crackers, chips, sweets, cookies, cakes, anything that you know is not healthy and if you drink pop, I am sorry to say that has to go out too. If you are like me you may find this task extremely difficult. However, it is in your best interest. If you cannot throw it out in the trash, give it to someone else who does not live with you or donate it to a food pantry. There are lots of them in need.

Over the years I have changed from eating regular yogurt to Greek yogurt which is better for you. I also swapped out skim milk for soy or almond milk. I changed from using vegetable oil to olive oil and now only use coconut oil. I hardly ever eat bread and when I do it is usually in the form of a tortilla wrap or flatbread. I have never really been a bread and butter person so it was not something that was real hard for me to give up. Meat was not difficult for me as my Mom had heart surgery several years back while I was still living at home and we changed our ways and started eating more and more chicken. Also, I eat tilapia, salmon and mild tasting fish. Variety is the spice of life and I agree so have been known to try new things out when I am out in a restaurant. I've always thought I would become a vegetarian as I love animals and do not like the idea of eating them, especially when I hear how poorly they are treated before being slaughtered. I'm still interested in making this change but for now I am putting it on the back burner.

As I said, I have tried a variety of diets, Weight Watchers, Slimfast, Richard Simmons, and have met with several dieticians and nutritionists too. I learned some new recipes but in the end the most important facts I think I learned is that I was not eating enough vegetables or drinking enough water. Weight Watchers taught me to drink enormous amounts of water as this helps fill you up and you should be drinking at least half your weight; in ounces of water . I am more apt to plan my meal around the vegetables I have as opposed to what my protein will be. Don't get me wrong as protein is very important and I have a lot of it throughout the day. It is just that most people do not realize how many vegetables make up a healthy food plan! I think the hardest thing for me to give up as far as protein goes, is cheese. Cheese is filled with all kinds of calories and I love the creamy taste of it! However, some of the lower fat cheeses are good and I like to experiment when it comes to food.

Constantly, I am trying out new recipes and experimenting with new foods. It happens that I get restless and bored with food so I like to vary what I eat. Therefore, I find myself looking for new ways to cook my meals and make them more exciting. However, I also know that sometimes very plain is the best way to go with your food.

Throughout the years, I have learned about food journaling, something that I do begrudgingly and I admit I am not faithful about this much needed tool. If you think you eat a healthy amount of calories in the day, try logging every single bite that goes in your mouth for a week and check to see how your caloric intake really is. Most people would be surprised that little tiny bite could add up to hundreds or even thousands of calories. Also, restaurants have started listing calories for some entrees, but check it out. Make the same thing at home and see if you get those same results. I tend to look at them as ballpark figures, not quite accurate calories. Also, do they add the bread into the meal or whatever other extras there may be?

HOW TO EXCEL AT WEIGHT LOSS AND BECOME MORE FIT AND HEALTHY

When I was growing up, Sunday dinner was a big thing in my house. It was a special family meal, usually started before church and we would come home to a nice smelling house. Mom was and still is a very good cook and also bakes delicious homemade desserts and treats. She never had a weight problem growing up and in fact was one of those people who were underweight and they wanted her to gain weight when she was in school! (In other words, the complete opposite of me.) Chips, cookies, candy, ice cream were all my friends while I was growing up! I could not get enough of them and they never let me down. Just like a kid in a candy shop, I could never leave these foods alone. I might miss out on something.

Socially, I felt like an outsider looking in... I was the last one chosen in gym class for teams, of course. I just felt socially awkward and my weight did not help. Of course, I remember those times in gym class when we got weighed in front of the whole class or ran through the Physical Fitness Tests. The only part I ever did well on was the sit ups and to this day, I love crunches and do them well. Remember those ugly gym uniforms we had to wear? I hated them and they made it impossible for me to hide my fat!

College of course, did not help me learn how to take care of myself. I was one of those who gained weight and actually in one year had accumulated 50 pounds extra on my body! I was homesick and did not enjoy it at all. I really did not know what I wanted to do with my life and all my friends were at home, not away at school. Therefore I quit after one year, knowing that someday I would go back to college somewhere and finish getting a degree. Luckily, being home was where I wanted to be and I was able to see my friends and thankfully the weight came off rather quickly.

It was later on that I started putting the pounds back on and then some. I know it is hard to believe that I did not notice but I never looked in the mirror as I did not like myself very much. I felt like a failure and acted like one too. Still remember how I woke up one day and was shocked to see all those pounds of flesh on my body! The bumps and lumps really got me and I started hating myself even more.

Now, looking back on this I can say I realize how negative I was back then. I have learned that you always have a choice in life. The glass is half empty or half full, as they say. The people who win in life are the ones who choose to be uplifting and positive every step of the way. Therefore it is important to work on your own emotions, feelings, belief and attitude in order to succeed on your weight loss journey. If you do not, you will either stop losing weight or gain it all back.

Taking time out every single day to do some kind of mindfulness activities is necessary. Meditation, journaling, centering, reiki, mirror work, yoga, deep breathing, and self-affirmation activities are all examples of exercises that will help you gain the right perspective about life. Physical movement and exercise are extremely important in helping me feel good and energized throughout my entire day.

 Sometimes I need to slow down the pace and check to make sure I am doing what is best for me, even if it is a cat nap in the middle of the day. I am the only one who is able to decide what is best for me and my body. If I am not taking care of my needs then I am "selling myself short". Would you want to buy a car that had been maintained well only half of the time? I know I would not.

None of us are perfect and we will not be able to maintain these goals all of the time. That is part of life and it is okay. However, each time you slip, try to become more and more conscious of your actions and the reasons behind your "slip". I will share an example here.

Years ago, I started exploring ways to deal with my binge eating disorder. I became involved in therapy sessions for them. One of the goals behind these sessions was to work on mindfulness about my thoughts, feelings, emotions and actions. What were the real reasons I was eating? Was I hungry, tired, sad, restless, or angry? What was going on the moment I started reaching for food? In exploring these actions, I realized a good amount of the time I was eating for the wrong reasons. Food is not really a friend and should only be used for nutritional substance, not to fill in an empty gap within your soul. Part of my discovery was how much food I would eat without any realization of it. Unconsciously I would reach for another bite, and another, and yet another, until the bag or box was empty. Somehow, I had to finish it and get rid of the evidence that the food ever existed!

Do you find yourself with a large bag of chips unopened and somehow the bag is empty in a matter of minutes, hours or even a day? Yet, you are the only one home? Then, you know exactly what I am talking about. To this day, I still have very good intentions when it comes to food but there are still some that I cannot be around as I lose control. However, I find that these "red light foods" can change from one day to the next. That is part of the reason I started exploring food labels, and how much sugar, salt, and fat content there is in each of these items.

For me, I know that artificial ingredients wreak havoc on my body. Sugar substitutes make me crave sugar even more than if I had none or even a little real sugar instead of the item. There have been studies that prove this too! That is the reason why the older I get, the closer I come to eating more raw and "clean" food. I have not done this 100% but it is in the works.

Processed food is full of chemicals and I believe cancer is caused by them. No one can tell me that it is a mystery that cancer runs rampant in our society today. When one ingredient like sugar for instance is decreased, then check and see if the manufacturer has increased the salt in that product. I know I have checked out peanut butter that is supposedly less fat or less sugar and have discovered the salt has been increased to make up for the taste! Therefore, I changed to natural peanut butter and even check these labels to make sure it really is just peanuts and oil blended without sugar or even cane sugar. Also, to combat this issue, I have even made some nut butters on my own and have discovered they are quite tasty!

The Dreaded "E" Word

If you are like me, you never played sports as a kid, were the last one picked in gym class for teams and hated physical fitness of any kind. You may have excelled at art, shop class, home economics, and choir or played an instrument in band or orchestra. Needless to say, any kind of physical activity was on the back burner for you and me alike. This was fine when we were kids, but as adults it is not. We need to be physically active in one way or another. It was not until I lost my Dad that I found true joy in an activity that is now recognized as exercise: namely Ballroom Dancing! It is through this flowing and freeing movement that I discovered the joy of dancing and losing all else to the beat and rhythm of the music. This was a brand new experience and felt so full of life to me. Somehow I could forget about everything else that was going on in my life and become one with the music and dance steps. I was on cloud 9!

Currently, I take Zumba classes and have revisited this joy of dance that is within my soul. In the future, I will become certified in this art form and teach classes to Senior citizens. When I miss my Zumba class for the week, watch out as you may encounter a bear.

Truthfully, my point is that it does not matter what you do to exercise as long as you do something. If I am limited to doing your normal average workout of pushups, sit ups, jumping jacks, etc. I soon become bored and ready to quit. Variety is the spice that holds me to an exercise program, without it I quit! Exercise makes some people energized right away but for me I do not always get this spark of adrenalin from it. However, I can definitely tell the difference the days that I do not exercise and the days that I do. My energy level is so much greater on the days that I have exercised or trained at the gym. Also, I am much more apt to be in a very good mood and even joking around with others on a good workout day. Without physical activity, I become a slug and have even noticed I do not think as clearly on these days.

Therefore, **find your passion**. Whether it is running, biking, boating, scuba diving, dancing; just get out there and do it. You owe it to yourself to feel the difference it can make in your life and it will also

help those pounds come off much easier.

Putting Life On Hold

Sometimes I feel like I have put my life on hold. I don't exactly know what I am waiting for as I

know this is not a dress rehearsal but the real thing. However, weight has a way of keeping me

from doing things; new adventures, risks, and travels that I would like to experience in my life.

How many times have you said, "I would do that if only I did not weigh so much?"

I remember the time I went white water rafting with a few friends. I actually only knew one other person on that trip and met the others on the way. I ended up driving, which was not planned but due to car problems. It was an interesting trip and it was fun. However, I remember talking to my friend beforehand about my embarrassment because of my

weight. Embarrassment and fear were mixed together and I was worried about being thrown

overboard and not being able to get back in the raft. I am glad I did not let these fears stop me from going on this trip, as it is the only time I have experienced white water rafting and I did

really enjoy it.

I will admit though, the one part of the trip that I did not like was when I jumped

off a cliff into the water and felt like I was drowning! It was scary enough but then once I finally

made it back to the raft; I had to have the guide pull me all the way back into the raft from the

water and that was very embarrassing. Of course, at that particular moment, I had better things

on my mind, like catching my breath for instance. Whew! Was I ever winded.

Why is it that we put things on hold? Shouldn't we find it necessary to take the bull by the horns, make the necessary changes to increase our health and lives and live fully, not limiting ourselves only to the things that are comfortable.

I cannot tell you how many times I need to remind myself about the internal limitations I have without even realizing it. Each time I go back to binge eating, I am limiting myself and reverting

back to the road I know, my comfort zone. However, challenge is what I need to find in each day in order to survive the way I crave to live my life: fully and wholly, as opposed to half-

heartedly. This is the reason that I never give up, no matter how many times I backslide, I keep

pushing to reach my goal. Now, you may say that it is going to take me longer than others to get there but I believe that I will be able to maintain my goal that much easier by taking the time to work through problems and things that are keeping me hidden behind the security my weight provides. Sometimes too, it is necessary to talk things out with a "life coach" or a counselor. Nobody should ever feel bad about needing some help to figure out the rough patches in life. The reason these people are there is to help others survive in this crazy fast world and help us figure out our roles in society as well as help us achieve the best possible attainment of our life goals, no matter what they may be.

It is time right now to take risks, adventure, walk, run and skip outside your comfort zone. Without doing this, you will never find out what living an abundant, full, exuberant life is all about. It is like a breath of fresh air.

29

I know I have said this before and I will say it again, Do not ever give up on yourself or your dreams. Give it all you got and you will make it! You are worth it!

COURAGE

The courage to take risks, moving into the unknown,

straying away from your comfort zone,

Seeing the boundaries and stretching beyond. Taking risks

to fulfill your dreams.

Standing proud like a lion when you feel like...

hanging your head

Roaring instead of whimpering...

Running instead of dragging your feet,

Shoulders up,   Chest out,   Smile planted on your face.

Keep going,   You got this....

Living....

It is worth the ride!

BONUS MATERIAL

I am thrilled to be able to include this passage in my book. It is

written by my current athletic trainer and I told him it was too good

not to share. Hope you enjoy it as much as I do!

BE A BIRD

As many of you know I have been on holiday for a few weeks and had a great time enjoying the weather in Florida. While it was hard for me to leave all of the valued connections that I am blessed enough to have made during my time here at Metro, it is equally important to stay connected to loved ones and recharge.

We started out our vacation plans with some sad news. We had plans to go back and spend some more time in Fiji, but about a week before we were scheduled to depart a natural disaster changed our thoughts of tropical paradise with the real probability of an emergency situation and evacuation. While we were disappointed at the cancellation of our destination, my wife and I had time already scheduled away from work and decided to drive to parts of Florida to visit friends and with a little luck get some sun and feel the comfort of sand between our toes.

This turned out to be one of the best vacations we have ever experienced! Because there was no agenda there were also no hotel reservations to keep and whatever direction we decided to take was the order of the day. Our only rule was to have fun! If we found for any reason that we weren't enjoying ourselves we simply moved on. This is different from most of the holidays that we have taken in the past and was a little hard to get accustomed to at first.

Then, as we were visiting Key West Florida we happened to notice something that normally would be ignored that helped put everything in perspective for us. Our realization came from a bird sitting in the sun on a log. We noticed how content this bird looked just taking in some sun; even though this bird could not sit in his spot forever it seemed as if he was serene enough to do just that. The bird eventually had to move, it just could not survive without food or shelter of some sort, however it had no concerns about these matters, and it was consumed only by the task at hand.

It occurred to me how much time, effort and anxiety that is expended anticipating the next thing that we will need to do to make things "perfect." The future is rarely perfect from our perspectives and will never be certain.

If we were to take this bird's example of how to live in the moment we might find that the "problems" that we are preparing for will never come. If those problems do eventually come and we have spent our time enjoying the "now" of our lives instead of fretting about the future we will likely have more energy to effectively deal with these issues when they actually occur.

Our holiday motto became "BE A BIRD." These simple words reminded us that the important things in life happen in an instant, THIS INSTANT.

I will continue to respect the important moments of my existence. "Right now" is the most precious gift that any of us will ever be able to enjoy.

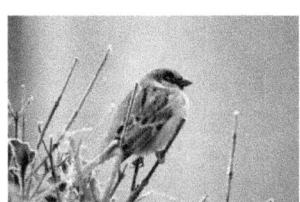

By: Keith Oliver

Special Thanks

I dedicate this book to a great guy, Dale L Roberts. You have supported me every step of the way and encouraged me to be true to myself. Without your support I would not have made it this far.

Special thanks to Mary Thibodeau for editing this book, Kelli Roberts for designing the cover and Dave Jackson for taking my picture! You each have given me the encouragement to share the real me with the world and I really appreciate it!

Keith Oliver, I must say thanks for sharing your wonderful writing ability. I am glad I can share this treasure with the world.

Special Gift to My Readers

For taking time to read my book, I would like to give you a **free resource** I have found helpful in losing weight. You can get it through this link! xlatw8loss.club

To my readers, I appreciate you taking the time out of your busy day to read my book. It would really help me out if you took a minute to tell me your thoughts, suggestions and comments about my writing. You can write a review on Amazon, which really helps authors become recognized worldwide and build their rankings! Here is my Amazon author page where you can find the rest of my collection:

http://www.amazon.com/Carol-Langkamp/e/B017WEFS8U

You can contact me at:

www.facebook.com/Carol.Langkamp.Readers/

www.cllsblogs.blogspot.com

Thank you and Have a Wonder-filled Day!

www.ingramcontent.com/pod-product-compliance
Lightning Source LLC
Chambersburg PA
CBHW071309280526
45788CB00004B/1862